COMPLETE GUIDE TO EOSINOPHILIC ESOPHAGITIS

A Comprehensive Handbook For Diagnosis, Treatment, Management Strategies, Essential Insights, Expert Guidance And Dietary Solutions

DEHART HAIRSTON

© [DEHART HAIRSTON], [2024]

All rights reserved. No part of this publication may be reproduced, distributed, or transmitted in any form or by any means, including photocopying, recording, or other electronic or mechanical methods, without the prior written permission of the publisher, except in the case of brief quotations embodied in critical reviews and certain other noncommercial uses permitted by copyright law.

DISCLAIMER

This book's content is only intended for general informative purposes. At the time of writing, the author has taken every precaution to guarantee that the material is correct and current. Nevertheless, the author disclaims all explicit and implicit representations and guarantees about the availability, appropriateness, correctness, completeness, and usefulness of the material on these pages.

Since the author is not a licensed medical practitioner, the material in this book shouldn't be interpreted as medical advice. Before making any modifications to their diet, exercise regimen, or medical treatment, readers are urged to speak with a licensed healthcare provider.

Moreover, the author has no connection to any of the businesses, organizations, or people that are discussed in this book. Any mentions of goods, services, businesses, or people are purely informative and do not indicate endorsement or suggestion.

This book's content is entirely dependent on the author's expertise, study, and comprehension of the topic. Despite having taken reasonable care to offer correct information, the author disclaims all liability for any mistakes or omissions in the material as well as for any losses, harm, or damages resulting from using the information.

It is recommended that readers use their own judgment and discretion when applying the knowledge in this book to their own situations. The use or implementation of any material in this book may result in unfavorable repercussions, directly or indirectly, for which the author assumes no liability.

By reading this book, you agree to release and hold the author harmless from any claims, losses, liabilities, costs, or expenditures resulting from or related to the use of the information you get from it.

Table of Contents

CHAPTER 1 11
    Understanding Eosinophilic Esophagitis 11
    What Is Eosinophilic Esophagitis? 11
    Causes And Risk Factors.......................................12
    Signs And Symptoms 13

CHAPTER 2 15
    Diagnosis 15
    Medical History And Physical Examination...........15
    Endoscopy And Biopsy 16
    Allergy Testing 17

CHAPTER 3 21
    Treatment Options 21
    Dietary Management 21
    Medications..23
    Allergen Immunotherapy 25
    Lifestyle Changes 26

CHAPTER 4 29
    Allergen Identification And Elimination 29
    Identifying Trigger Foods.....................................29
    Elimination Diets 30

Food Allergy Testing 31
CHAPTER 5 35
　Medications 35
　Corticosteroids 35
　Proton Pump Inhibitors (Ppis) 37
　Immunomodulators 40
　Biologic Therapies 42
CHAPTER 6 45
　Dietary Management 45
　Elemental Diet 45
　Elimination Diets 47
　Food Texture Modification 49
　Nutritional Supplements 50
CHAPTER 7 53
　Lifestyle Modifications 53
　Eating Habits And Meal Timing 53
　Positioning During And After Meals 55
　Stress Management Techniques 56
CHAPTER 8 59
　Managing Symptoms 59
　Addressing Dysphagia 59

Dealing With Heartburn 61
Preventing Food Impaction 64
CHAPTER 9 67
Long-Term Management And Follow-Up 67
Regular Monitoring 67
Adjusting Treatment Plans 69
Pediatric Considerations 71
CHAPTER 10 75
Living Well With Eosinophilic Esophagitis 75
Support Groups And Resources 75
Coping Strategies 77
Advocacy And Awareness 79
CONCLUSION 82
THE END 85

ABOUT THIS BOOK

"Eosinophilic Esophagitis: A Comprehensive Guide to Understanding and Managing Your Condition" is a must-have resource for anybody living with eosinophilic esophagitis (EoE) or caring for someone who has it. EoE is a chronic, immune-mediated esophageal illness that may have a major effect on a person's quality of life. This book is a light of information, providing insight, advice, and practical answers for navigating the challenges of EoE.

In Chapter 1, readers learn about the principles of EoE, including its existence, causes, and the vast range of symptoms it exhibits. This fundamental understanding is essential for detecting and successfully treating the illness. Chapter 2 includes critical information on identifying EoE, such as the importance of medical history, physical examination, endoscopy, biopsy, and allergy testing, allowing patients to seek prompt and correct diagnoses.

Chapters 3–6 are the core of the book, delving deeply into numerous therapy approaches. Readers learn how to successfully treat EoE via food management and pharmaceutical alternatives, as well as allergy detection and elimination tactics. This holistic approach allows patients to personalize their treatment regimens to meet their specific requirements, resulting in improved symptom management and general well-being.

Furthermore, Chapters 7 and 8 include practical advice and tactics for making lifestyle changes and managing symptoms daily. By covering topics such as eating habits, meal scheduling, stress management, dysphagia, and heartburn, this book provides readers with the skills they need to overcome the difficulties of EoE with confidence and resilience.

Chapter 9 focuses on long-term management and follow-up, highlighting the significance of frequent monitoring and making changes to treatment programs over time. This proactive approach guarantees that people can monitor their status and make educated health choices.

Finally, Chapter 10 provides a comprehensive overview of living well with EoE, including resources, support groups, coping skills, and advocacy campaigns to help people flourish despite the problems they experience. In essence, "Eosinophilic Esophagitis" is more than just a book; it is a lifeline for individuals suffering from this ailment, providing hope, empowerment, and a path to a better quality of life.

CHAPTER 1

Understanding Eosinophilic Esophagitis

What Is Eosinophilic Esophagitis?

Eosinophilic esophagitis (EoE) is a chronic inflammatory illness affecting the esophagus, the muscular tube that links the neck and stomach. It is characterized by the accumulation of eosinophils, a kind of white blood cell, in the esophagus tissue. These eosinophils may trigger inflammation, resulting in symptoms and serious consequences.

The actual etiology of EoE is unknown, however, it is thought to be an aberrant immunological reaction to certain foods or environmental allergens. When someone with EoE consumes certain triggers, it may cause inflammation in the esophagus, leading to the symptoms associated with the illness.

Causes And Risk Factors

While the exact etiology of EoE is unknown, various variables may contribute to its development. Genetics are likely to have a part since EoE runs in families. Individuals with certain gene variants may be predisposed to developing the illness when exposed to particular environmental triggers.

Food allergies and sensitivities are highly associated with EoE. Dairy, wheat, eggs, soy, and shellfish are some of the most common triggers. Elimination diets, which exclude certain probable allergens from the diet, are often used as part of the diagnostic and therapy process to identify and control trigger foods.

Environmental allergens such as pollen, dust mites, and pet dander may further aggravate EoE symptoms in some people. These allergens may cause an immunological response, resulting in inflammation in the esophagus and increasing symptoms such as trouble swallowing, chest discomfort, and heartburn.

Other risk factors for EoE include a history of allergies including asthma, eczema, or allergic rhinitis (hay fever). Furthermore, EoE is more frequent in men and usually appears during youth or early adulthood, but it may happen at any age.

Signs And Symptoms

The signs and symptoms of EoE vary according to the individual's age and the severity of the ailment. Symptoms in newborns and young children may include difficulty eating, low-weight growth, vomiting, and stomach discomfort.

Older children and adults with EoE often have difficulties swallowing (dysphagia), which may result in food impaction. Other typical symptoms include chest discomfort, heartburn, regurgitation of food or saliva, and recurring instances of food becoming lodged in the esophagus.

Esophageal strictures, or narrowings of the esophagus caused by persistent inflammation and scarring, are one of the consequences of EoE. These strictures may cause chronic difficulties swallowing and may need endoscopic dilatation to expand the esophagus.

It is critical to identify the signs and symptoms of EoE and get medical attention if you or your kid exhibits any alarming symptoms. Early diagnosis and treatment may help people with EoE manage their symptoms, avoid complications, and improve their quality of life.

CHAPTER 2

Diagnosis

Medical History And Physical Examination

Eosinophilic Esophagitis (EoE) is normally diagnosed after a comprehensive medical history and physical examination. Your healthcare professional will inquire about your symptoms, when they began, how often they occur, and if anything seems to cause them. It's important to be as descriptive as possible during this conversation since it will assist your doctor in identifying probable reasons and rule out other disorders with comparable symptoms.

During the physical exam, your doctor will most likely concentrate on your throat and abdomen. They may check for evidence of inflammation or other abnormalities that suggest EoE.

However, it is crucial to remember that a physical examination alone cannot establish a diagnosis of EoE; further testing is often necessary for a clear diagnosis.

Endoscopy And Biopsy

Endoscopy is an important diagnostic technique for EoE. An endoscopy involves inserting a thin, flexible tube with a camera at the end (known as an endoscope) into the mouth and the esophagus. This enables the clinician to visually examine the esophagus for evidence of inflammation, constriction, or other abnormalities consistent with EoE.

Biopsy is often used during endoscopy to confirm the presence of eosinophils in the esophagus. Eosinophils are white blood cells that cause allergic responses and inflammation. In individuals with EoE, eosinophils are often seen in greater numbers than normal in the esophageal tissue. During the biopsy, tiny tissue samples are removed from the esophageal lining using specialized tools inserted via the endoscope. These samples are then analyzed under a microscope for eosinophils and other inflammatory markers associated with EoE.

It is critical to follow any pre-endoscopy advice given by your healthcare professional, such as fasting before the operation. Endoscopy is a relatively safe operation, although there are certain dangers, such as hemorrhage or esophageal perforation, but these problems are uncommon.

Allergy Testing

Because EoE is often related to food and environmental allergies, allergy testing may be required as part of the diagnosis procedure. Allergy testing may help identify particular allergens that may be irritating the esophagus.

Skin prick tests, blood tests (such as specific IgE testing), and elimination diets are some of the allergy testing techniques available. Skin prick tests include applying tiny quantities of allergens to the skin and then pricking or scratching it to check whether a response develops. Blood tests detect the amount of particular antibodies generated in response to allergens. Elimination diets entail eliminating probable trigger items from the diet for some time before returning them to evaluate whether symptoms improve or worsen.

It is important to collaborate closely with your healthcare physician to select the best allergy testing approach for your needs. Allergy testing results, together with other diagnostic findings, may be used to guide therapy options and management strategies for EoE.

Healthcare experts may diagnose EoE and design an effective treatment plan suited to your specific requirements by carefully reviewing your medical history, doing a comprehensive physical examination, performing an endoscopy with biopsy, and perhaps undertaking allergy testing. Early diagnosis and therapy are critical for treating EoE and increasing the quality of life for people with this illness.

CHAPTER 3

Treatment Options

Dietary Management

Dietary control is critical in the treatment of Eosinophilic Esophagitis (EoE), since some foods may cause inflammation in the esophagus. The initial step in dietary management is frequently to identify and eliminate trigger foods using an elimination diet. This entails eliminating common allergies such as dairy, wheat, soy, eggs, nuts, and shellfish from the diet for a period of six to eight weeks. During this period, symptoms are evaluated to see which meals are triggering the inflammation.

Following the elimination phase, foods are reintroduced one at a time to determine particular triggers.

To guarantee safety and efficacy, this technique is carried out under the supervision of a healthcare expert, such as an EoE-certified dietician. Once trigger foods have been identified, they are permanently eliminated from the diet to avoid flare-ups.

In addition to avoiding trigger foods, some people with EoE may benefit from a particular diet known as the six-food elimination diet. This diet eliminates the six most prevalent triggers: dairy, wheat, soy, eggs, nuts, and seafood. It is often used when normal elimination diets do not effectively reduce symptoms.

Working with a dietician may be quite beneficial for people who struggle to adhere to dietary restrictions. They may provide advice on meal planning, recipe adjustments, and eating-out techniques that adhere to dietary restrictions. It's crucial to remember that dietary management isn't a one-size-fits-all solution and may need continuing modifications to get the best symptom relief.

Medications

Medications are another key component of treating Eosinophilic Esophagitis, and they are often used in combination with dietary changes. Medication treatment aims to decrease inflammation and relieve symptoms such as trouble swallowing, chest discomfort, and heartburn.

Proton pump inhibitors (PPIs) are a frequent kind of drug used to treat EoE. These drugs limit stomach acid production, which may help relieve symptoms and facilitate esophageal repair. PPIs are often used as a first-line therapy and may be beneficial in certain cases with mild to moderate EoE.

In addition to PPIs, corticosteroids may be administered to minimize esophageal inflammation. These drugs may be taken orally or applied topically via a swallowed steroid inhaler. Topical steroids are generally favored over oral steroids because they have less systemic negative effects.

Individuals with severe or refractory EoE may benefit from biologic medicines. These drugs target immune system components that contribute to the inflammatory response. Biologics are often reserved for patients who do not react to conventional treatments or who have severe adverse effects from standard therapy.

As with any medicine, you must carefully follow your healthcare provider's instructions and quickly report any adverse effects or concerns. Furthermore, drug therapy may need to be modified over time depending on symptom intensity and treatment response.

Allergen Immunotherapy

Allergen immunotherapy, commonly known as allergy injections, may be advised for people with Eosinophilic Esophagitis who have identified particular dietary or environmental allergens as causing their symptoms. This therapy includes progressively exposing the immune system to small doses of the allergen to desensitize the body's reaction over time.

An allergist often administers allergen immunotherapy in the form of injections or sublingual drops. The treatment period might run from several months to years, depending on the individual's reaction and the severity of their allergies. While allergen immunotherapy has been demonstrated to be useful for illnesses such as allergic rhinitis and asthma, its function in treating EoE is currently under investigation.

Allergen immunotherapy is still considered an experimental treatment for Eosinophilic Esophagitis and is not generally accessible. However, research in this area is continuing, and future studies may provide light on its potential advantages and limits in controlling EoE.

Lifestyle Changes

In addition to food control, medicines, and allergy immunotherapy, lifestyle adjustments may help manage and alleviate symptoms of Eosinophilic Esophagitis. These adjustments might consist of:

• Elevating the head of the bed helps avoid acid reflux and esophageal discomfort.

• Avoid wearing tight clothes, especially around the waist, since it may exert pressure on the stomach and raise the risk of acid reflux.

• Eating smaller, more frequent meals might reduce stomach distention and strain on the esophagus, perhaps preventing symptoms of EoE. Eating smaller meals more regularly might assist in relieving pressure and discomfort.

• Managing stress: Relaxation, mindfulness, and therapy may help alleviate symptoms of Eosinophilic Esophagitis.

• Tobacco and alcohol use may aggravate symptoms of EoE and increase the risk of acid reflux. It is recommended to avoid both.

Individuals with Eosinophilic Esophagitis may benefit from implementing these lifestyle adjustments into their daily routine, resulting in better symptom management and general health. It is critical to collaborate closely with your healthcare physician to create a complete treatment plan that covers all parts of the problem.

CHAPTER 4

Allergen Identification And Elimination

Identifying Trigger Foods

Identifying trigger foods is a critical step in treating Eosinophilic Esophagitis (EoE). These are meals that trigger an allergic response in the esophagus, resulting in inflammation and symptoms such as trouble swallowing, chest discomfort, and heartburn. Identifying trigger foods requires a methodical process of observation, removal, and reintroduction.

To begin, maintaining a comprehensive food journal might give useful insights. Documenting what you eat and any resulting symptoms might help you identify trends and possible trigger foods. It's critical to be precise, documenting not just the major components but also spices, sauces, and cooking techniques.

Once probable trigger foods have been identified, an elimination diet may be suggested. This is eliminating potential allergens from your diet for a certain length of time, usually under the supervision of a healthcare practitioner or qualified dietitian. During the elimination phase, it is critical to avoid all potential triggers to precisely analyze their influence.

Elimination Diets

Elimination diets are organized strategies for identifying and eliminating trigger foods that contribute to EoE symptoms. exclusion diets may be approached in a variety of ways, including elemental diets, single-food exclusion, and multiple-food elimination.

Elemental diets entail taking just amino acid-based formulas for a certain length of time, giving adequate nutrition while removing any possible allergies. This procedure is often employed in extreme instances or when other approaches fail.

Single-food elimination diets remove one putative trigger item at a time, allowing for close monitoring of symptom improvement. Common trigger foods include dairy, wheat, soy, eggs, nuts, and shellfish. Elimination usually lasts a few weeks to a month, with regular monitoring of symptoms.

Multiple-food elimination diets include the exclusion of numerous putative trigger foods at the same time. This strategy is more thorough but needs careful attention and may demand the assistance of a healthcare expert to guarantee nutritional sufficiency.

Food Allergy Testing

Food allergy testing may supplement dietary treatments by giving objective information about possible trigger foods. However, it is critical to recognize the limits of these tests and interpret the findings in light of clinical symptoms.

Skin prick tests and blood testing, such as IgE antibody tests, may detect particular IgE antibodies generated in reaction to allergens and so diagnose immediate-type food allergies. However, EoE is largely caused by delayed-type hypersensitivity responses, which may not always result in positive allergy testing.

Endoscopic methods, such as esophageal biopsy, are the gold standard for diagnosing EoE and may also detect dietary allergen-induced inflammation. During an endoscopy, tiny tissue samples from the esophagus are collected and tested for eosinophilic infiltration, which provides direct evidence of inflammation.

In certain circumstances, allergy elimination diets may be guided by allergy testing findings, which may assist in prioritizing foods to exclude. However, negative allergy testing may not rule out the potential of food triggers, since EoE might entail immune responses that are not IgE-mediated.

Overall, a comprehensive strategy that includes dietary change, symptom monitoring, and, where applicable, food allergy testing is critical for successfully treating EoE and identifying trigger foods unique to each person. Close coordination among patients, healthcare professionals, and dietitians is required to enhance nutritional regimens and improve outcomes for people with EoE.

34

CHAPTER 5

Medications

Corticosteroids

Corticosteroids are an important component in the therapy of Eosinophilic Esophagitis (EoE) since they diminish inflammation in the esophagus. These drugs may be given orally, topically (via inhalers), or intravenously, depending on the severity and scope of the illness.

Oral corticosteroids, such as prednisone or budesonide, are often given for short-term usage to relieve symptoms during flare-ups. These drugs act by inhibiting the immunological response, which reduces eosinophil infiltration in the esophagus and relieves symptoms such as trouble swallowing, chest discomfort, and heartburn. However, long-term use of oral corticosteroids is typically discouraged owing to the possibility of serious side effects such as weight gain, osteoporosis, and increased susceptibility to infection.

Topical corticosteroids, such as inhalers or sprays, are sometimes used as a maintenance treatment for EoE. These drugs are administered directly to the esophagus, usually by swallowing or gargling, and may help decrease inflammation and prevent symptoms from recurring. Budesonide, in particular, is often used in this way owing to its local anti-inflammatory properties and decreased systemic absorption, which reduces the danger of systemic adverse effects associated with oral corticosteroids.

Intravenous corticosteroids may be reserved for severe cases of EoE or when oral or topical therapies have proven unsuccessful. Intravenous corticosteroids are administered in a clinical environment and give immediate symptom alleviation by administering large dosages of drugs straight into the circulation. This technique, however, is often reserved for short-term treatment because of the risk of major side effects and the necessity for regular monitoring by healthcare specialists.

While corticosteroids may be very useful in managing symptoms and inflammation in EoE, they must be used with caution and under the supervision of a healthcare expert to reduce the risk of side effects and provide the best therapeutic results.

Proton Pump Inhibitors (Ppis)

Proton Pump Inhibitors (PPIs) are a kind of drug that is often used to treat acid-related illnesses such as gastroesophageal reflux disease (GERD), as well as Eosinophilic Esophagitis (EoE). These drugs act by inhibiting proton pumps in the stomach lining, lowering stomach acid production, and relieving symptoms such as heartburn and acid reflux.

While PPIs may not directly address the underlying inflammation that causes EoE, they can help reduce symptoms associated with acid reflux, which can increase esophageal inflammation and pain in people with EoE. PPIs, by lowering the acidity of stomach contents that reflux into the esophagus, might help reduce tissue damage and irritation, possibly complementing existing anti-inflammatory therapy for EOE.

Omeprazole, lansoprazole, and esomeprazole are examples of commonly prescribed PPIs. They are usually given orally as capsules or tablets. These drugs are often used as first-line therapy for EoE, either alone or in conjunction with other therapies, depending on the patient's symptoms and illness severity.

In addition to their function in treating acid reflux symptoms, PPIs may offer anti-inflammatory characteristics that might assist people with EoE.

Some studies show that PPIs may help lower esophageal eosinophilia, albeit the mechanism is not entirely understood. As a result, PPIs may have a dual therapeutic function in EoE, targeting both acid reflux symptoms and underlying inflammation.

However, it is crucial to emphasize that, although PPIs may help many people with EoE, they may not give full symptom relief or disease management on their own. As a result, they are often used as part of a complete treatment plan that may include other medicines, dietary changes, and lifestyle adjustments to properly control the illness.

Immunomodulators

Immunomodulators are a kind of drug that alters or regulates the immune system's response, making them potentially effective in the treatment of immunological-mediated illnesses such as Eosinophilic Esophagitis (EoE). These drugs target particular immune system components to lessen inflammation and the aberrant immunological response that causes EoE.

Azathioprine, a thiopurine, is a popular immunomodulator used in the treatment of EoE. Azathioprine acts by limiting the growth of immune cells engaged in inflammation, lowering the generation of inflammatory mediators, and regulating the immunological response in the esophagus.

Methotrexate, a folate antagonist that interferes with DNA and RNA synthesis, may also be used to treat EoE by reducing immune cell proliferation and inflammation. Methotrexate is often reserved for those with severe or refractory EoE who have not responded to previous therapies since it has a greater risk of adverse effects and needs thorough monitoring by doctors.

Immunomodulators such as azathioprine and methotrexate are often utilized as second-line or supplementary treatments for EoE, especially when corticosteroids or proton pump inhibitors have proven ineffective or poorly tolerated. These drugs may be given for long-term use to assist in maintaining remission and avoid illness recurrence, although their effectiveness and safety profiles may differ across people.

While immunomodulators may help manage inflammation and symptoms in EoE, they may also have adverse effects such as bone marrow suppression, liver damage, and increased susceptibility to infection. As a result, persons taking immunomodulators must undergo continuous monitoring and follow-up with their healthcare providers to achieve optimum treatment results and reduce the risk of unwanted effects.

Biologic Therapies

Biologic treatments are a newer class of drugs that target particular molecules involved in the immune response, providing a more tailored approach to treating inflammatory illnesses such as Eosinophilic Esophagitis (EoE). These drugs are generated from live creatures or created using technological methods and are intended to disrupt particular processes or proteins involved in the pathophysiology of EoE.

Monoclonal antibodies that target interleukin-5 (IL-5), a cytokine that regulates eosinophil production and activation, are one of the most promising biological therapies for EoE. By inhibiting IL-5 activity, these biological treatments may limit the recruitment and activation of eosinophils in the esophagus, hence reducing inflammation and symptoms associated with EoE.

For example, mepolizumab and reslizumab are monoclonal antibodies that target IL-5 and have been demonstrated in clinical studies to reduce esophageal eosinophilia and improve symptoms in people with EoE. These drugs are usually given as subcutaneous injections at regular intervals and may be used as a maintenance treatment to help avoid illness recurrence and sustain remission.

Dupilumab, a biologic drug targeting IL-4Rα, a critical mediator of type 2 inflammation, has shown potential in treating EoE. Dupilumab, which blocks the IL-4Rα pathway, may improve symptoms and histologic findings in persons with EoE by reducing esophageal inflammation and modulating the immune response.

Biologic treatments provide the benefit of focused therapy while possibly causing less systemic adverse effects than typical immunosuppressive drugs such as corticosteroids or immunomodulators. However, they are often more costly and may need frequent monitoring and administration by healthcare personnel, restricting their availability to certain people with EoE.

Overall, biologic medicines are a promising improvement in the treatment of EoE, providing new alternatives for those who do not respond to traditional treatments or have major adverse effects. More research and clinical studies are required to better understand these drugs' long-term effectiveness and safety, as well as their appropriate role in the treatment of EoE.

CHAPTER 6

Dietary Management

Elemental Diet

An elemental diet is like resetting your digestive system, particularly if you have Eosinophilic Esophagitis (EoE). Consider a diet in which you ingest just the most basic, easy-to-digest nutrients in liquid form. This method relieves your esophagus from coping with potentially irritating meals.

So, what is on the menu? Consider elemental formulae to be the superhero version of nutrition; they include all of the important amino acids, lipids, carbs, vitamins, and minerals your body needs to operate, but in a form that requires minimum digestion. This implies less labor for your digestive system, allowing your esophagus time to recover.

It is not always easy to implement an elemental diet. It takes dedication and frequently means saying goodbye to typical meals over some time. However, the benefits may be enormous, particularly for people dealing with EoE symptoms. Giving your esophagus a vacation from possible triggers allows it to heal and minimize inflammation.

Doctors sometimes prescribe beginning with a rigorous elemental diet for a specified amount of time, usually a few weeks. During this period, you will only eat elemental formulae and avoid all other meals and beverages. It's like pausing your normal diet and allowing your body to reboot.

Let us now discuss the practical aspects. Elemental formulations come in a variety of forms, including powders, ready-to-drink liquids, and semi-solid choices. Your healthcare professional will advise you on the best choice based on your specific requirements and preferences. Some individuals find it useful to flavor formulations with extracts or syrups to make them more appealing. And remember, hydration is essential, so drink lots of water throughout the day.

Elimination Diets

Elimination diets are similar to playing detective with your food. What's the goal? Identify and remove any possible triggers that may be exacerbating your EoE symptoms. These triggers may differ from person to person, making it something of a trial-and-error procedure. But don't worry, with time and advice from your healthcare team, you can identify which items are causing problems and eliminate them from your diet.

So, how does this work? Well, it begins with a thorough examination of your diet and symptoms. Your healthcare physician may advise you to maintain a food diary to note what you eat and any associated symptoms. This information is very helpful in identifying possible triggers.

Once you've compiled a list of questionable items, start removing them one by one. This enables you to examine how different foods impact your symptoms. Keep in mind that symptoms may take some time to improve after eliminating a trigger meal, so patience is required.

Elimination diets may be beneficial, but they are not without obstacles. Cutting off some foods might be difficult, particularly if they are mainstays in your diet. Furthermore, there is always the potential of unintentionally eliminating essential nutrients. That's why it's critical to collaborate with your healthcare physician or a qualified dietician during the procedure.

Once trigger foods have been identified, the next step is to devise a long-term eating plan that avoids them while still supplying all of the nutrients your body needs. This may include finding substitute items or cooking techniques to replace the omitted meals.

Food Texture Modification

Food texture adjustment aims to make mealtimes easier on your esophagus. Certain textures may elicit symptoms such as trouble swallowing or chest discomfort in people with EOE. Modifying the texture of meals makes them simpler to swallow and less likely to irritate your esophagus.

So, what exactly does texture modification entail? It may include anything from chopping, blending, or pureeing meals to achieve smoother textures. Think soups, smoothies, or soft, mashed foods. These softer textures are kinder to the esophagus, making them simpler to swallow and less prone to irritate.

However, texture adjustment is more than simply softening meals; it is also about avoiding potentially troublesome textures. Crunchy or scratchy meals, such as raw vegetables or rough meats, may be difficult to swallow and may worsen EoE symptoms.

Texture adjustments may need some imagination in the kitchen, but the results are worthwhile. Making modest modifications to the texture of your meals allows you to eat a larger range of foods without pain or trouble swallowing.

Nutritional Supplements

Nutritional supplements provide a safety net, ensuring that you obtain all of the critical nutrients your body requires, particularly when dietary limitations are in place due to illnesses such as EoE. These supplements come in a variety of formats, including vitamins and minerals, protein powders, and meal replacement drinks.

Nutritional supplements may help persons with EoE maintain their health, particularly if specific food categories are off-limits owing to trigger foods. Supplements may help cover nutritional gaps and ensure that your body receives all of the critical elements it needs to operate normally.

However, not all supplements are made equal, so it's important to pick intelligently. Your healthcare physician or a certified dietitian may assist you in picking the appropriate supplements depending on your specific requirements and dietary limitations. They may also guarantee that you are taking supplements in safe and effective quantities.

When adding vitamins to your regimen, consistency is essential. Take these exactly as advised, and keep track of how you feel afterward. If you encounter any side effects, see your doctor.

In addition to typical supplements, there are specialist formulae made exclusively for those who have EoE. These formulations are often hypoallergenic and devoid of typical trigger components, making them safer choices for those with food sensitivities.

By adding nutritional supplements into your daily routine, you may improve your general health and well-being, even if you have food limitations due to disorders like EoE. Just remember to check with your doctor before beginning any new supplement regimen to verify it is safe and suitable for you.

CHAPTER 7

Lifestyle Modifications

Eating Habits And Meal Timing

Eating habits and meal timing are critical for controlling eosinophilic esophagitis (EoE). Simple changes to your diet and meal pattern may help relieve symptoms and improve your overall quality of life.

To begin, consider any items that may increase your EoE symptoms. These triggers differ from person to person, but they often include dairy, gluten, soy, eggs, and specific fruits or vegetables. Keeping a food journal might help you identify which meals cause pain and avoid them in the future.

In addition to avoiding trigger foods, eating at regular intervals may help reduce flare-ups.

To lessen the pressure on your esophagus, eat smaller, more frequent meals rather than larger ones. Eating slowly and chewing deeply may also help digestion and reduce irritation.

Meal time is another factor to consider. Refraining from eating too close to bedtime may help reduce acid reflux and discomfort when sleeping. To ensure good digestion, eat your final meal at least two to three hours before sleep.

Furthermore, eating a balanced diet rich in whole grains, lean meats, fruits, and vegetables may improve overall gastrointestinal health and minimize esophageal inflammation. Experimenting with various cooking techniques, such as steaming or baking, may make meals more digestible and less likely to cause symptoms.

By making these dietary changes and paying attention to meal scheduling, you may successfully control your EoE symptoms while enjoying meals without pain.

Positioning During And After Meals

Proper posture during and after meals may have a substantial influence on your experience with eosinophilic esophagitis (EoE). Simple postural modifications might help to alleviate discomfort and improve digestion.

One effective method is to sit upright while eating. Avoiding slouching or laying down when eating may help keep food from regurgitating into the esophagus, lowering the risk of discomfort and inflammation. Sitting on a comfortable, supportive chair with your back straight will help you maintain appropriate alignment and swallow more easily.

After meals, staying upright for at least 30 minutes may help digestion and avoid acid reflux. This enables gravity to help move food down the digestive system, reducing the probability of food remaining in the esophagus. Light physical exercise, such as a brief stroll, might aid digestion and relieve pain.

Additionally, raising the head of your bed helps reduce overnight reflux and alleviate nocturnal symptoms. Using bed risers or putting blocks under the legs of the bed frame may provide a small inclination, preventing stomach acid from running back into the esophagus while sleeping.

By using these posture strategies, you may enhance your digestion, decrease reflux, and reduce inflammation in the esophagus, resulting in more overall comfort and well-being.

Stress Management Techniques

Stress management is critical for people with eosinophilic esophagitis (EoE), since it may aggravate symptoms and cause flare-ups.

Incorporating relaxation methods into your daily routine may help reduce stress and enhance esophageal healing.

Deep breathing exercises are an efficient stress-management method. Deep breathing may stimulate the body's relaxation response, which reduces stress hormone production and calms the neurological system. Find a quiet, comfortable place to sit or lie down, shut your eyes, and take long, deep breaths, concentrating on the feeling of air entering your lungs and then slowly leaving them.

Mindfulness meditation is another effective way to manage stress and improve emotional well-being. Mindfulness meditation, which cultivates present-moment awareness and nonjudgmental acceptance, may help you deal with the difficulties of living with a chronic disease such as EoE. Begin with small sessions of five to ten minutes and progressively increase the time as you get more comfortable with the exercise.

Regular physical exercise, such as yoga or tai chi, may also help decrease stress and increase resilience. These mind-body techniques combine mild movement and breath awareness to promote relaxation, flexibility, and inner calm.

In addition to these approaches, finding healthy ways to express feelings, such as writing, creative arts, or chatting with a trusted friend or therapist, may help you manage stress.

By adding stress management practices into your daily routine, you may lessen the influence of stress on your EoE symptoms while improving your general quality of life.

CHAPTER 8

Managing Symptoms

Addressing Dysphagia

Dysphagia, or difficulty swallowing, is a common symptom of Eosinophilic Esophagitis (EoE) that may have a substantial influence on one's quality of life. Managing dysphagia requires a multifaceted strategy suited to the individual's requirements.

First and foremost, identify trigger foods that may increase dysphagia symptoms. Common triggers include dairy, gluten, soy, eggs, and some fruits and vegetables. Keeping a food journal may assist in identifying these triggers, allowing for more focused dietary changes.

In addition to dietary adjustments, a variety of swallowing procedures may be used to alleviate dysphagia symptoms.

These might include eating smaller meals, chewing deeply, and washing each mouthful down with lots of water. Some people find that eating softer foods or pureed meals helps them swallow more comfortably.

Furthermore, using relaxation methods like deep breathing or mindfulness might help minimize the anxiety associated with dysphagia. Anxiety and worry may worsen swallowing issues, therefore controlling these emotions is critical for symptom treatment.

For those with severe dysphagia, speech therapy may be needed. Speech therapists may teach exercises and procedures to enhance swallowing function while lowering the risk of choking or aspiration.

If dysphagia continues after dietary and lifestyle changes, medical treatment may be required. This may involve using oral steroids to lessen inflammation in the esophagus or performing dilation operations to enlarge constricted regions of the esophagus.

Regular follow-up with a healthcare practitioner is critical for monitoring symptom development and adjusting treatment techniques as required. Dysphagia associated with EoE may be successfully controlled by using a holistic strategy that addresses dietary, lifestyle, and medical issues, enabling people to have better swallowing function and overall quality of life.

Dealing With Heartburn

Heartburn, which causes a burning feeling in the chest or throat, is a typical symptom of Eosinophilic Esophagitis (EoE) and may be quite uncomfortable. Managing heartburn requires a mix of food adjustments, lifestyle changes, and, in some circumstances, medical treatment.

One of the first stages in treating heartburn is to identify trigger foods that may aggravate symptoms. Acidic foods and drinks including citrus fruits, tomatoes, coffee, and alcohol are all common causes. Spicy foods, fatty meals, and big servings may all lead to heartburn. Keeping a food journal may assist in identifying these triggers, allowing for more focused dietary changes.

In addition to food adjustments, lifestyle improvements may help relieve heartburn symptoms. These may include not laying down just after eating, raising the head of the bed when sleeping, and keeping a healthy weight. Smoking cessation is particularly important since it may aggravate acid reflux and raise the risk of problems.

Over-the-counter antacids and acid reducers may give brief relief for heartburn symptoms. However, for those who have chronic or severe heartburn, prescription drugs such as proton pump inhibitors (PPIs) may be required to limit stomach acid production and relieve symptoms.

When medical treatment fails to relieve heartburn, surgical surgery may be considered. Fundoplication is a procedure that helps strengthen the lower esophageal sphincter and prevents stomach acid from refluxing into the esophagus.

Regular follow-up with a healthcare practitioner is critical for monitoring symptom development and adjusting treatment techniques as required. Heartburn caused by EoE may be successfully controlled by using a holistic strategy that addresses dietary, lifestyle, and medical variables, enabling people to have better symptom management and overall quality of life.

Preventing Food Impaction

Food impaction, or the obstruction of the esophagus by food particles, is an unpleasant consequence of Eosinophilic Esophagitis (EoE) that needs immediate treatment. Preventing food impaction requires a mix of dietary adjustments, lifestyle changes, and proactive actions to reduce the risk of blockage.

One of the most important measures for reducing food impaction is to identify and eliminate trigger foods that may cause esophageal constriction or inflammation. Bread, pork, and fiber fruits and vegetables are among the most common trigger foods. Keeping a food journal may assist in identifying these triggers, allowing for more focused dietary changes to lower the risk of impaction.

In addition to dietary improvements, changing eating behaviors may reduce the risk of food impaction. This may involve taking smaller pieces, chewing deeply, and eating slowly to avoid huge food boluses being trapped in the esophagus. Avoiding eating when preoccupied or in a hurry may also assist with effective chewing and swallowing.

Individuals with a history of food impaction may benefit from esophageal dilatation treatments, which enlarge restricted sections of the esophagus. These treatments may help lower the risk of impaction while also alleviating symptoms including dysphagia and chest discomfort.

Regular follow-up with a healthcare practitioner is critical for monitoring symptom development and adjusting treatment techniques as required. In certain circumstances, regular monitoring of endoscopies may be indicated to examine the esophagus mucosa and identify symptoms of constriction or inflammation.

Food impaction caused by EoE may be successfully avoided with a holistic strategy that addresses dietary, lifestyle, and medical issues, enabling people to experience better symptom management and overall quality of life.

CHAPTER 9

Long-Term Management And Follow-Up

Regular Monitoring

Regular monitoring is required to appropriately manage eosinophilic esophagitis (EoE) throughout time. This includes scheduled appointments with healthcare providers to assess the condition's progress and the efficacy of the treatment plan. These sessions are typically held every few months, however this might vary based on individual circumstances.

During these monitoring visits, several elements of the patient's health are assessed. Symptoms are one of the primary focus areas. Patients are advised to mention any changes or new symptoms they have had since their previous visit. Healthcare providers may also inquire about any issues or difficulties with the current treatment regimen.

In addition to symptom assessment, healthcare providers may use diagnostic tests to determine the level of inflammation in the esophagus. This frequently includes an endoscopy with biopsy, in which small tissue samples are taken from the esophageal lining and examined under a microscope for the presence of eosinophils, the signature immune cells associated with EoE.

Regular monitoring serves several functions in the management of EoE. It enables healthcare providers to track the disease's progression, evaluate the efficacy of current treatments, and make any necessary changes to the treatment plan. It also allows patients to ask questions, express concerns, and seek support from their healthcare team.

Adjusting Treatment Plans

Because EoE is a chronic condition, treatment plans may need to be adjusted over time to ensure the best management of symptoms and inflammation. The decision to change treatment is made based on several factors, including the patient's response to current therapies, the severity of symptoms, and changes in disease activity.

Medication management is a common treatment plan adjustment. Depending on the patient's response, healthcare providers may adjust the dosage of medications like proton pump inhibitors (PPIs), swallowed steroids, or other anti-inflammatory drugs. If the current regimen is ineffective in controlling symptoms or inflammation, alternative medications may be prescribed.

Dietary changes are another aspect of treatment plans that may require modification. Patients with EoE frequently use food elimination diets to identify and avoid trigger foods that aggravate symptoms. Reintroducing eliminated foods and monitoring reactions over time can help to fine-tune the diet plan. Healthcare providers may also recommend consulting with a dietitian to ensure that nutritional requirements are met while adhering to dietary restrictions.

In addition to medications and dietary changes, patients with esophageal strictures or narrowing may benefit from endoscopic dilation. This procedure can help to relieve dysphagia (difficulty swallowing) and improve esophageal function.

Regular communication between patients and healthcare providers is critical in determining when treatment adjustments are required. Patients should promptly report any changes in symptoms or disease activity so that their treatment plan can be modified as needed.

Pediatric Considerations

Pediatric patients' unique developmental and nutritional needs necessitate special considerations when managing EoE. Treatment approaches for children may differ from those used in adults, and healthcare providers must consider factors such as growth and development, dietary preferences, and the child's ability to follow treatment regimens.

To confirm the diagnosis of EoE, pediatric patients may undergo similar diagnostic procedures to adults, such as an endoscopy with biopsy. However, the interpretation of symptoms and test results may differ depending on the child's age and communication skills.

Pediatric patients may benefit from a multidisciplinary approach to treatment, which includes pediatric gastroenterologists, allergists, dietitians, and other specialists as needed. This team-based approach ensures that each child receives comprehensive care that is tailored to their specific needs and circumstances.

Dietary management is frequently a cornerstone of EoE treatment in pediatric patients. Elimination diets, in which specific food triggers are identified and removed from the child's diet, are widely used to treat symptoms and reduce inflammation. However, implementing dietary restrictions in children can be difficult and may necessitate constant monitoring and support from parents or caregivers.

To control inflammation and symptoms, pediatric patients may be prescribed swallowed steroids, proton pump inhibitors, or other medications.

Healthcare providers must consider medication dosage and formulation based on the child's age, weight, and ability to swallow pills or capsules.

Regular follow-up appointments are essential for monitoring the child's growth, development, and response to therapy. Pediatric patients may require more frequent monitoring and changes to their treatment plan as they grow and their nutritional requirements change.

In summary, managing EoE in pediatric patients necessitates a personalized approach that takes into account the child's specific needs and circumstances. Collaboration among healthcare providers, parents, and caregivers is critical to improving treatment outcomes and ensuring the child's well-being.

CHAPTER 10

Living Well With Eosinophilic Esophagitis

Support Groups And Resources

Living with eosinophilic esophagitis (EoE) might be lonely, but you are not alone. Support groups and resources are important while negotiating the hardships of this disease. Joining a support group, either in person or online, may help you connect with individuals who understand what you're going through. These communities enable you to share your experiences, ask questions, and receive support from individuals who understand the difficulties of EoE.

Online forums and social media groups devoted to EoE give essential information and support. There are strategies for managing symptoms, assistance in handling food limitations, and support from those going through similar circumstances.

Furthermore, many organizations and charities devoted to EoE provide online resources, instructional materials, and forums where you may contact professionals and other patients.

Beyond internet assistance, consider about joining local support groups or attending EoE-related activities in your region. Meeting people in person may help you create deep ties and develop a feeling of community. These groups typically host instructional sessions, guest speakers, and social events that give both support and education.

In addition to support groups, there are several resources available to aid you in understanding and managing EoE. Books, blogs, podcasts, and online courses give vital information on the disorder, treatment choices, and coping skills. Medical practitioners who specialize in EoE may also give individualized counsel and assistance depending on your unique requirements.

Coping Strategies

Living with EoE demands resilience and adaptation. Coping skills may help you overcome problems and retain a positive mindset. Education is one of the most effective coping mechanisms. Understanding the origins, symptoms, and treatment options for EoE allows you to take control of your health and make educated choices.

Managing stress is crucial for general well-being, particularly when living with a chronic disease like EoE. Practices such as mindfulness, meditation, and deep breathing exercises may help decrease tension and promote relaxation. Finding things that offer you pleasure and relaxation, whether it's spending time with loved ones, pursuing hobbies, or appreciating nature, may also be excellent for your mental and emotional health.

Developing strong communication skills is vital for navigating the problems of EoE, especially when it comes to advocating for your needs with healthcare professionals, family members, and employers. Learning how to assertively communicate your concerns, ask for assistance when required, and establish limits will enable you to properly manage your illness and maintain a healthy lifestyle.

Dietary control has a crucial role in treating EoE symptoms. Working with a licensed dietitian or nutritionist who specializes in EoE may help you design a tailored eating plan that reduces symptom triggers while maintaining sufficient nutrition. Keeping a food journal to monitor symptoms and identify possible triggers may also be useful in managing your diet properly.

Finally, building a strong support network of friends, family, and healthcare professionals is vital for managing EoE. Surrounding yourself with others who understand and support you may give emotional validation, practical aid, and encouragement during tough times. Remember that it's all right to ask for support when you need it, and that you don't have to endure EoE alone.

Advocacy And Awareness

Advocacy and increasing awareness are key components of living well with EoE. By sharing your experience and educating others about the illness, you may help decrease stigma, boost understanding, and encourage support for EoE patients and their families. Advocacy may take numerous forms, from participating in awareness events and fundraisers to sharing informative information on social media.

One of the most potent ways to advocate for yourself and others with EoE is by being an active member of the EoE community. Joining advocacy groups and organizations devoted to EoE enables you to contribute your voice to key concerns, support research initiatives, and lobby for legislative changes that benefit EoE sufferers.

Raising awareness of EoE in your neighborhood and abroad is another key advocacy technique. Hosting educational events, distributing instructional materials, and connecting with local media sources may assist enhance knowledge and exposure of the illness. By sharing your experiences and ideas, you may help others identify the signs and symptoms of EoE and support early identification and intervention.

In addition to promoting awareness among the general public, pushing for increased access to healthcare and treatment choices is crucial for ensuring that EoE sufferers get the care they need. This may entail lobbying lawmakers, engaging in advocacy campaigns, and supporting efforts that attempt to enhance healthcare services and resources for EoE sufferers.

By being an advocate for yourself and others with EoE, you can help establish a more supportive and inclusive environment for everyone impacted by this illness. Whether it's via raising awareness, offering information, or pushing for legislative changes, your actions may make a substantial impact on the lives of EoE patients and their families.

CONCLUSION

In conclusion, Eosinophilic Esophagitis (EoE) is a complicated and increasingly recognized chronic inflammatory condition of the esophagus. Throughout this research, it has become obvious that EoE offers considerable hurdles in diagnosis, treatment, and understanding its underlying processes. While the specific reason remains uncertain, it is commonly believed that both genetic predisposition and environmental variables contribute to its development.

Diagnostically, the gold standard is now endoscopic biopsy revealing eosinophilic infiltration of the esophagus mucosa, however, non-invasive approaches are under development. The treatment of EoE often requires a multidisciplinary approach, including dietary change, medication, and mechanical dilatation in refractory patients. However, there is an urgent need for new effective, and focused therapy choices, particularly for patients who do not react to present medications or have major adverse effects.

Research into the pathogenesis of EoE has emphasized the significance of immunological dysregulation, allergy reactions, and genetic vulnerability. As such, current research is concentrating on unraveling these pathways to uncover potential therapeutic targets and biomarkers for better disease management and personalized treatment.

Furthermore, EoE profoundly damages patients' quality of life, with symptoms ranging from dysphagia and food impaction to reduced social functioning and psychological discomfort. Therefore, comprehensive treatment that treats both the medical and emotional elements of the illness is vital.

In conclusion, although significant progress has been achieved in understanding and controlling EoE, several problems exist. Collaborative efforts among doctors, researchers, patients, and advocacy organizations are vital to further our understanding, strengthen diagnostic skills, optimize treatment regimens, and ultimately improve outcomes for persons living with EoE.

THE END

www.ingramcontent.com/pod-product-compliance
Lightning Source LLC
Chambersburg PA
CBHW070315230526
45470CB00002B/880